I0448343

Note for Librarians: A cataloguing record for this book is available from Library and Archives
Canada at www.collectionscanada.ca/amicus/index-e.html
ISBN 1-4120-6849-5

*Printed on paper with minimum 30% recycled fibre. Trafford's print shop
runs on "green energy" from solar, wind and other environmentally-friendly power sources.*

TRAFFORD
PUBLISHING™

Offices in Canada, USA, Ireland and UK

This book was published *on-demand* in cooperation with Trafford Publishing. On-demand
publishing is a unique process and service of making a book available for retail sale to the
public taking advantage of on-demand manufacturing and Internet marketing. On-demand
publishing includes promotions, retail sales, manufacturing, order fulfilment, accounting and
collecting royalties on behalf of the author.

Book sales for North America and international:
Trafford Publishing, 6E–2333 Government St.,
Victoria, BC v8t 4p4 CANADA
phone 250 383 6864 (toll-free 1 888 232 4444)
fax 250 383 6804; email to orders@trafford.com

Book sales in Europe:
Trafford Publishing (uk) Limited, 9 Park End Street, 2nd Floor
Oxford, UK ox1 1hh UNITED KINGDOM
phone 44 (0)1865 722 113 (local rate 0845 230 9601)
facsimile 44 (0)1865 722 868; info.uk@trafford.com

Order online at:
trafford.com/05-1760

10 9 8 7 6 5 4 3 2

light

joy

love

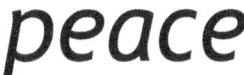

peace

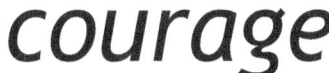

courage

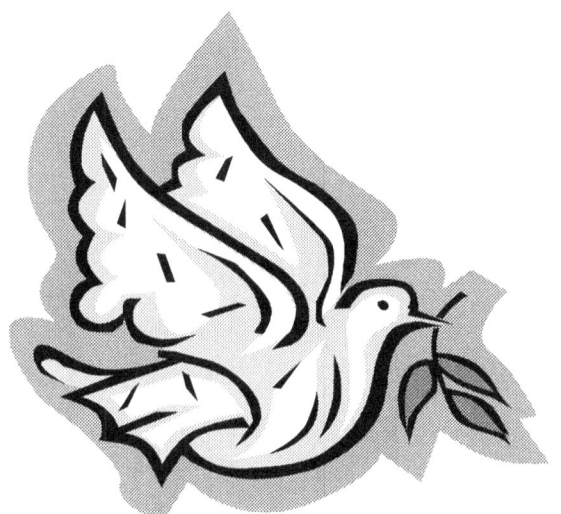

DEDICATION

I wish to dedicate this book to my children - Philip, Nathan, Adrienne, and Kathleen. May they experience to the fullest, the absolute joy of the human journey on the Earth as we all step up into the frequencies of the fourth dimension!! To my Creator who channeled this through me so patiently and so graciously, no words can express our gratitude for the gifts in knowledge that these pages contain! Gifts that ensure our very survival and our upliftment! Love and Light to you all!!

Donna Boynton

INDEX

INTRODUCTION

In the Earth's creation there was considerable planning. In the beginning the Earth was a pristine, uninhabited space, free of pollutants, of noise, of stressors. This has all changed as you are all sadly aware. These changes from the original environment have taxed the human body a hundredfold. No longer can the liver of your bodies discard the toxins that beset them. No longer can the spleen metabolize the bewildering array of chemicals and compounds that comprise your food and drink. No longer can the lungs breathe in the quality of air they require to serve the fire of the heart-the furnace of your bodies. No longer can the kidneys strain out the harmful bacteria that infest your drinking waters.

I am providing the necessary information now to assist your bodies. First is their improvement to the status of health in this polluted environment using only those valuable food resources still available. Further to that, in subsequent books, I will advise on the techniques, the foods, the resources you must use to facilitate the body's rise in frequencies. For as I write this, the frequencies that orchestrate your entire universe are now changing upward.

This means that all of Planet Earth - her microbes, her bacteria, her germs, her plants, her animals, her trees, and her humans will be forced to metabolically adjust to these rising frequencies. In light of the widespread imbalances presently existing, this will spell disaster in some areas and joy in other areas as the multiplication of some organisms will cease, yet others will increase.

I cannot recommend enough to you the implementation of these instructions, these recipes, these pieces of information. For the original plan of the Earth's evolution did contemplate a time when higher frequencies would lead to ecstasy - that is in a balanced Earth system.

This is your manual for restoring balance within your body-and therefore the world. For your bodies are of this world and do reflect this Earth's health. As each of you addresses these issues in your own body you do address this world wide issue. The care of your bodies is incredibly important!!

I begin with an understanding of the energy transfer system of the human body. This will enable you to digest this information more readily. It will enable you to see the necessity of these teachings I deliver. There is within each cell a storehouse of energy awaiting a command from the systems of the body. For example, in the liver, millions of cells are at the ready to build new red blood cells. When a command, via a chemical from the brain, is delivered to the cell, it begins much as a factory, to work in concert with many other cells to manufacture these red blood cells. These red blood cells deliver oxygen, nutrients, even enzymes to the various sites of the body for repair, rebuilding, even the body's very propulsion in the physical world, its' eating, sleeping, playing, working.

From this one simple structure, the individual cell, all processes are built. To enable this energy release, the cell requires two components-water and salt. Without these, death of the individual cell and finally the entire body would ensue. For when a body dies it is the withdrawal of the salt from the cells that does occur. Verify this by checking the fluids departing the body at this time.

So to enhance the cell mechanism, water and salt are critical. It is so because you originated from the seas in your evolution. Now, 75% of your bodies are still composed of this saline solution. So when either the water or the salt is deficient, so too is the energy transmission of the body. To improve the energy of the body immediately, pay heed to your water and salt consumption. This is number one!

However the quality of these two components is becoming

increasingly even more important to your body's delivery of energy. As your water quality diminishes, so too will the functioning of the body

In these pages I address the quality of the water and how to improve it quickly. I address the salt you are presently using and the terrible detractions it visits on your bodies. And finally I address the very fuel, via food, that you are providing your bodies.

This food-fuel is the wood in the furnace, so to speak. Once the furnace -each cell- is working efficiently then what remains is the wood you choose to burn in the furnace. Certain foods will deliver higher BTUs per burn than others obviously- a hot dog versus a steak, a soda pop versus orange juice.These food choices are next in importance in the energy delivery system.

The surroundings, the activities, even the wearing apparel also affect the healthy energy delivery system of your bodies. I do stress that you are very compromised in these areas - of salt and water, of energy delivery –whether to fight cancer, invading microbes and bacteria or the common cold. However with the ever rising frequencies besetting your planet, the necessity of developing an even more efficient energy delivery system in the body looms.

For as these frequencies rise, the body will be subjected to ever higher frequencies that do indeed fuel the very energy exchange in your bodies. Higher demand will be put on your very cells to produce more energy to survive-even thrive- in these new frequencies. To step into these higher frequencies as you all must, major considerations are required.

This then is the topic of these pages that follow. Remember-I am your Creator. Your well being is indeed my concern!!

IONIZED WATER

A key factor contributing to the absorption of nutrients by the body's blood system is the ionization of the water consumed. The body is 75% water. All cellular activity is dependant on maximum hydration. Six to eight glasses of the highest quality water is absolutely essential.

The term ionization refers to the balance of negative and positive ions in a substance-in this case the drinking water. When negative ions are low, the salts in the body can not conduct energy across the cell wall. With the lack of "energy" or electrical spark, the minerals in the digesting food will not bind to the cells in the body. They will instead be excreted from the body in urine, perspiration, or in the respiration. Lost valuable nutrients!

You can test your home water supply to determine the % of negative ions to positive ions. A balanced state-equal negative and positive- is optimum. For the test you need:

- *1 tsp. iodized salt*
- *1 tsp. natural vinegar*
- *3 Tbsp. of water to be tested*
- *1 tarnished copper penny*

Mix the first three ingredients together. Let stand for 3 minutes. Add the tarnished copper penny. See chart below;

If the penny becomes shiny and bright:

- *Within 3 minutes - water is 80% +ve ions to 20% -ve ions.*
- *Within 2 minutes - water is 70% +ve ions to 30% -ve ions.*
- *Within 1 minute - water is 50 % +ve to 50% -ve.*

To remedy the % ionization of your water to 50% -ve and 50% +ve, you need 500 gauss magnets with a true North and true South. These are available at craft stores and hardware stores. Use a compass to determine the North side. Mark this North side with a marker.

Tape the North side of the required number of magnets to the side of the container you use for your drinking and cooking water:

- 1 litre container - 500 gauss - Takes 5 minutes to ionize
- 4 litre container - 1000 gauss - 10 min.
- 10 litre container - 3000 gauss - 2 hours
- 50 litre container - 4000 gauss - 2 hours
- 60 litre container - 5000 gauss - 2 hours
- 100 litre container - 10000 gauss - 2 hours

Water that is balanced in negative and positive ions tastes different. It is "alive" to the taste buds. It has a vibrant charge. When you cook foods in balanced ionized water, nutrients are retained, flavour enhanced. The nutrients are readily absorbed by the body's cellular structure which itself is 75% water. It takes about 30 days of drinking this improved water to restore the fluids in the body to the balanced ion state.

Coated pills, medications, vitamin and mineral supplements do not dissolve well in either balanced ionized water or unbalanced. Which leads you to consider.... what is actually happening to that coated tablet in your body with its' 75% water composition?

ACID-ALKALINE BALANCE

Integral to the body's ability to source the minerals and the vitamins in your food supply is balance in a state called the acid-alkaline environment. Imbalanced acidic conditions in the body leave it vulnerable to parasitic invasion as well as viral and bacterial invasions. Inflammations, diseases you describe as an "itis"- that is dermatitis, colitis, neuritis etc. thrive in an acid environment, not to mention the existence of pathogens such as tape worms and larvae.

Alkaline environments facilitate the growth of Candida, a fungus, which debilitates entire systems in the body.

Alkaline implies overly sweet and acid implies overly sour. Neither condition fosters wellness. This scale indicates the acid-alkaline level balance in the body:

10	Highly Alkaline
9.0	
8.5	
8.0	
7.4	At 7.4 the body is in balance. A slightly alkaline environment is required for maximum nutrient uptake by the body.
7.0	
6.5	
6.0	
5.5	
5.0	Highly Acid

To test your body's acid-alkaline balance, a simple test can be conducted. Put 200 ml of fresh water in a clear glass container. Add 1 drop of pure iodine. When you first urinate in the morning, save 1 Tablespoon of the urine to mix with the iodine –

water mixture. Let stand 10 minutes. Shake it up. Then check the colour against the following chart to determine the reading.

Violet	9.0
Indigo	8.5
Blue	8.0
Red	7.4
Yellow	7.0
Orange	6.5
Cloudy white	6.0
Black (grey)	5.5

Readings between 7.00 and 7.4 are acceptable. Your body is sourcing the trace minerals if your diet contains those necessary trace mineral and key vitamins. See recipe selections given. This is a simple home test. The results are not warranted. For the purposes of this book it will suffice.

Consult your medical doctor if extreme conditions appear to exist. To restore the acid-alkaline balance see the chart below:

9.0	No wheat products-breads, pastas, crackers, cookies etc,(corn meal and rice are allowed) for 5 days
8.5	3 large organic oranges a day, eaten together, for 5 days *see note
8.0	3 large organic oranges a day eaten together for 5 days **see note
7.4	Normal
7.0	1 lemon squeezed into 8 oz water with ½ tsp iodized sea salt first thing before breakfast for 3 days
6.5	1 lemon squeezed into 8 oz. water with ½ tsp iodized sea salt before breakfast for 5 days
6.0	1 lemon squeezed into 8 oz water with ½ tsp iodized sea salt before breakfast for 7 days ***see note

Note!! In the alkaline treatments no other fruit is to be eaten throughout the 3 days.

*** Note!! If oranges are not tolerated substitute each orange with ½ cup pure organic cranberry juice.*

*** *Note!! In the acid condition no extra salt should be consumed in the days listed.*

SALT

The next component on your earth that causes considerable distress is common table salt. This salt you consume at meals has been altered to make it whiter, make it pour easier, make it dissolve on the taste buds quickly to prompt the desire for more.

Salt-original salt-is very valuable to the electrolytic processes in the body's cells. That is the transmission or reception of the electrical charge from negative to positive depends on the saline nature of the body tissues. To overcome the additives of your common table salt it is necessary to revisit the actual function of this precious salt. These additives in fact prevent the transmission of electrical impulses across the cell wall-the very purpose in the first place!! So replace the common table salt with iodized sea salt-the best substitute at present for the real thing!

I cannot stress enough how important the mineral composition of this good salt is to your body! With the ever increasing, higher frequencies there is acceleration in the electrical charges attempting to cross the cell walls in the body. This good salt is the very key to your survival in these times ahead!

I also ask you to reconsider the excessive use of salt on your roads in winter as this salt is finding its way into plant tissues and waterways. This further diminishes nature's ability to move to these new frequencies. In turn she fortifies your bodies with the necessary nutrients for your spiral upward in evolution. You must now see how it is all "one"! You are what you eat! If the plant or animal you consume also has the impoverished state caused by these excess items in your food supply so too will you be impoverished. So replace all salt with iodized sea salt immediately to see an improvement in the essential mineral status of the body.

AS I SEE IT!!

When preparing fruits and vegetables for your consumption, I advise you to bathe them in your ionized water plus 1 Tbsp of natural vinegar. This will rid the produce of any harmful effects from their growing, handling or transportation.

For the vegetables you do not peel, immerse them in their bath for upwards of 10 minutes. Then dry off and store in the refrigerator. I must advise that the life (that is, the nutrient's life) of these vegetables is very short. I recommend the process of lacto-fermentation to increase the nutrients available and also the purchase of small quantities of vegetables at a time. All vegetables may be washed together.

In the case of fruits, bathe these separately as some do not like the company of others and will cause more rapid spoilage. I again recommend the preserving of these fruits as given to extend their time of value.

If your drinking water is not balanced in negative and positive ions, the white sugar you ingest sits in the stomach undigested. To remove it before it putrefies, the body releases chemical substances that rely on minerals for their composition, to break down the sugar. This depletes the body's mineral reserves to the extent that there are few left to do the essential work in the body-such as building enzymes, digesting proteins and fats. This also leaves the body weakened and vulnerable as it has no reserves to protect itself in times of bacterial or viral invasion.

The necessary nutrients have been allocated to breaking down the inert white sugar in the stomach. Sugar cane has its own supply of natural enzymes to aid in its digestion. I say it is a "live" food. So in the body it adds to the nutrients. It does not deplete the body's reserves. Cooking with sugar cane as a substitute for refined white or brown sugar will give the body immediate relief from nutrient depletion.
Fruit sugars are also difficult to digest particularly in an acid/alkaline imbalance in the body. The fruit sugars ferment in

the stomach causing gas to build up. Fruit fermented in vodka-for a few days facilitates the breakdown by the body and increases the nutrients available to the body for its essential needs.

In the matter of spelt, it is a type of wheat that I highly recommend due to its' ionization. That is... it is high in negative ions. This means it is able to attract enzymes to facilitate its breakdown in the body. Other grains such as ordinary wheat, rye, oats, buckwheat are not charged as high negatively as spelt is. It therefore takes much longer for the body to digest and to attract the essential nutrients that the grain itself holds in store.

This is why the breads, cakes and cookies you are now consuming of regular wheat products are so demanding on the body's nutrient reserves. Lessen the demand through the choice of spelt flour and once again you immediately release more essential nutrients into the body's store. This is the objective: to fortify the body-nutrient wise for growth, repair, maintenance and trouble shooting when bacteria, virus, protozoa and Candida- whatever, attempts to invade the system. This will become a major concern shortly. I cannot emphasize this enough! The level of health, shall I say body protection against these forces is at the lowest level ever in the entire history of mankind. This is hard to believe in face of the so- called progress, parts of your planet enjoy. But it is so and I am here now to provide recourse to this dire situation.

I now address the use of sugar in your food supply. Though it sets a craving for more, it is in fact lowering all of the body's systems in an effort to digest it as stated previously. Furthermore there is a compound in white sugar that leaches out key enzymes that manufacture the necessary building blocks for proteins and for protein synthesis in the body.

Thus the consumption of so much sugar leaves the body defenseless to the aforementioned invaders - the Invaders of the Lost Ark - the ARK being the human body - shall I say!! You are much improved in stature when you choose to consume honey, *raw sugar cane, molasses, or maple syrup for those especially in Northern areas who have access to this nature's food straight from the earth herself!*

I now offer you the subject of oils. Sunshine imparts energy to the earth, to you, to all that lives and grows on the earth. So consuming the fruits or the oils of that which grows on the earth imparts this frequency of high energy once again to your bodies. The body enjoys this energy many times over when you consume the fruits, nuts, and oils of the plants and trees.

I can not emphasize enough the value of these sun ripened products to uplift and enliven your wellbeing here on Mother Earth. These are gifts available to you daily for your consumption and enjoyment.

To be specific, sunflower seed oil has a very high frequency. This is because of those bright yellow petals that the flower sports. Yellow attracts such a high frequency band of energy. This is imparted to the seed that grows so prolifically in the centre of the flower. Evidence of this vast storehouse of energy is the very height the sunflower plant achieves in one short growing season. Take note how other yellow flowering plants also obtain greater height or density or profusion due to this same mighty vibration it is attracting from the sun. So if you want energy eat crushed sunflower seeds or the oil of the sunflower. I am emphatic when I say that it is your energy savior!!

Grow sunflowers everywhere to attract this energy to your gardens, your fields, your parks, your Earth!!

So now I turn to the issue of nuts such as walnuts, hazel nuts, brazil nuts and almonds – even peanuts, though not as good a source of energy and overused in an oily spread on starchy white bread. Better to reach for the whole peanut in the shell- unprocessed and thereby avoiding the reduction in negative ions caused by over processing of nature's products. For you see the processing of any natural food be it plant or animal does diminish the negative ions available to the body. And remember it is the negative ions that are attracted to enzymes that the body produces as "attractors" for its' continuing sustenance

You are not finite. You are infinite! So the body, though it is merely flesh and bone must also strive now in these new frequencies, those of the fourth dimension, to become infinite!! No easy task as it is presently being fuelled with such low frequency food with little or no negative ions.

Now to the nuts! Again Nature requires very high frequencies of light to produce the "fruit" of her trees and plants-that is the height of the summer when the sun is strongest. So these frequencies are imparted to the resulting "fruits" that is nuts. This creates yet another incredible source, for you to tap into these "summer time" frequencies, over and over again each time you consume the nut-be it brazil, almond hazel etc. That is why at the lowest time of earth's reception of life giving energies for you in the Northern climates, in late December the Christmas nuts in the shell are available. You need their goodness most around the shortest day of the year. So eat up!! Nature is there to assist your well being, nay even your "exaltedness" shall I say!! It is about upliftment in the grandest sense! If the body can rise into these new frequencies as I suggest it can indeed, it will only be done through the enhancement of your foods. So eat nuts, especially from the shell, when first they come off the tree.

The oils I speak of also impart this frequency to your body when ingested. There are ways of using each oil that are important. Sunflower seed oil should not be heated as in frying, as it loses its high frequencies rapidly. Choose instead to put it in your salads, your cakes, cookies, breads as you are mixing in the dry ingredients and the wet. That way a synergy is occurring between the ingredients that allow all of the goodness of the sun's frequencies to come forth. I emphasize the value of your sunflower seed oil!

Though there is no brazil nut oil, there is the mighty brazil nut itself! Chew on these often as they are ripe with frequencies that will sustain your body through this incredible shift in energy. Stockpile your brazil nuts so you may enjoy them though others will not see their value. They will sustain you I declare!!

Black walnuts are particularly attracting to all the sun's frequencies so eat these in abundance as well. I use them in many of the recipes in place of the flour. This will impart even higher frequencies to your breads, cakes, and cookies. And rightly so!! You are here to enjoy the earth and her gifts, her bounty.

Though almonds in skins are better for you, their skin has tannin that is disagreeable to the stomach acids. So I recommend that you soak these almonds in skins in ionized water plus iodized sea salt to rid them of this tannin: One cup of almonds, one cup of water and one tsp. of salt for two hours. Drain, then spread out on a baking sheet and slow roast in a 250 degree oven for several hours. Then enjoy!! They are also a storehouse or veritable power plant of energy. Add a little iodized sea salt to them in the drying phase to enhance them .I am aware of the need to feed the taste buds and the "sight" buds when preparing and eating food. These are also a part of the gifts I speak of.

Now to the use of corn oils and canola oils. Though these plants grow on earth's surface attracting frequencies from the sun they are not convertible to oils that are compatible with the enzymes of the human body. So I recommend a very limited use of these oils if any use at all. Better choices are sunflower seed, hazel nut, grape seed and of course the mighty olive - king of oils!!

The olive I have left to last. As you say "save the best for last"! Grown in Southern climates where the sun's intensity is greatest, it captures the most of the valuable frequencies your body so desperately needs from now on to survive. For I am speaking of survival here-as well as "thrival"-new word! Start using it!! You all deserve to thrive! The tools are here. Use them for your "thrival"!

The olive's oil is so potent - or so full of "potent-ial' that I stress its' use in cooking, baking, barbequing, sautéing. I recommend at least three Tbsp. a day as your daily requirement whatever the body size or age. This can be hidden in salads, supper dishes, baked goods, however you can cleverly apply it. You can even apply it to your skin to protect and lubricate it. Revel in it!! Olives are "olive-it"! (Pun here. Who said I am always serious?)

Now on to the butter that comes from your bovines. This oil or "fat" as you call it is for the maintenance and sustenance of your body as well as the mighty olive. It imparts a special oil that can only come from the bovine-who through digestion of nature's plants creates an enzyme that you need to break down very specific, yet necessary[necessary is an understatement here] for the body's energy needs. There is a combination here that I call "synergy" that enables the body to tap into resources that it could not otherwise. This is more important than you presently know to the mental faculties of the human being. Infants also need to acquire this nutrient or "factor X' as Weston Price called it. So new mother's eat butter, drink milk, then breastfeed your babies for their acceleration into these new higher frequencies. You are responsible for their passage forward to experience this epoch of "thrival"!

As for the merits of honey, bees skirt around and dance with the flowers. Flowers are frequencies. See all the colours they produce as a feast for the eyes in summertime. The bees simply taste, in a sensual way, the results of this high frequency within the plant structure that is the product pollen. With this pollen dusting on its legs, the bee move from flower to flower doing a sexual dance for all the flowers. In so doing the bee captures the vibration of all these flowers.

Their colours are the true reflection of the life giving frequencies coming directly from the sun- frequencies that you can not yet see as colour. So the bees impart these frequencies to the honey they produce in their hives. You harvest the honey, then spread it on negatively ionized spelt bread, ingest it and continue the dance of the sensual in every cell in your body, long after the sun's high frequencies have departed from winter's blast.

So use honey to sweeten your breads, cakes, cookies, then arouse once again, the senses in your body! This is your playground. Sense it to the fullest! Where do you go from here? To heaven!! The ultimate in delights!

I will now address the topic of flower as in flowers of the fields. Herbs are your best friends shall I say. They are aromatic to the extent that they attract vibrations to your sense of smell, the nose - a very important vehicle - for receiving vibrations of wellness or health. These plants were designed for your evolution- dare I say, your "revolution" into higher states or frequencies!

Basil is the king of the plant world! So sad it requires a hot climate to grow at its best. Again this bares witness to the high vibration it captures in its fragrant leaves. These leaves are best used when absolutely fresh as their vibration will then enhance your vibration maximally. Use them in soups, salads, even in breads. Buy them when they are young seedlings. Place them on your window sills as even then they will be transmitting their vibrations into your living spaces for your bodily needs.

This is well known among those who live in the Mediterranean, an area of the world most prolific in foods that are high in energy, So use basil everywhere, in everything!
Mint is also a plant you can have in your homes and on your properties. Any variety will enhance the absorption of those energies necessary to sustain growth and aliveness for your physical bodies. I say this even as you are thinking it will run rampant if left uncontrolled. That is so! So keep it confined to a pot or a container on your patios and decks. This "rampant" nature attests to its voracious acceptance of these frequencies that expedite growth and development-the very factors required by the human body as it strives to move into a finer and finer state of being now in these climates of higher frequencies that have beset the earth.

I know you are now beginning to understand the signs that a plant is a conduit for these energies or frequencies by their growth habits. Think about those plants that love to ramble or invade as you say and realize their metabolism has been accelerated by the very frequencies of the sun beaming on the earth, Common grass grows so fast you invented mowers to keep it at bay so you could see above it. Know that surrounding your houses with grass is a good thing as it imparts energy to every step you take on it. I know you are aware of the aesthetics of your place but do allow these "ramblers" to have their place as they provide great service to you in health in the summer months.

There is a danger that your weed killers will eliminate the very plants that offer to sustain you through this time of great upheaval for the physical body. Do practice allowance. Let the aesthetics be in the array of ramblers that wish to take up residence near you- the dandelion as well! These are harbingers of the new energy working through you to take you to shall I say "ecstasy"! Who would equate a dandelion with ecstasy? See the sunny yellow face and know that is what awaits you as you step up to these new frequencies! Dandelions!! But seriously, they portend what joy awaits as the body's frequencies accelerate to the levels it is attempting to reach. Give it the tools that already wish to support your wellbeing-ness on this planet Earth!

Now to the leaves on the trees. In the spring they are small, fresh green in colour. This green guides the juices or sap of the human body-by frequency- to cleanse the cellular structure. It is a quickening frequency so the effect it has is to quicken the movement of fluids through the cellular structure thus cleaning and sweeping out the debris of winter. So bathe your eyes in this colour by frequent walks in green forests where every leaf is beckoning to your body to turn on the "self-cleaning" switch for its yearly maintenance. Do not sit indoors when this very miracle of the physical world awaits you!

Other areas of this world do not have this "self-cleaning" mechanism available to them and must rely on potions and

*elixirs to do this tremendously important job. Nor do they have
your winters that beset the body with considerable stress that
does create more "debris" to be removed in the spring "clean-
up"! This is the double edge of living in the Northern climates.
But I say to you this also has its benefits.*

*The white of your snows and the barren, darkness of your trees
are elixirs in their own right. They stimulate the mind to
thoughts of compassion and higher insight. These vibrations
create a contrast of frequencies that stimulate a reflective
approach to the turmoil of the world. Be not so quick to judge
the goings on as good or bad rather as a conundrum for the
human being to handle. That is the value of winter to the
human spirit as I see it, through frequencies imparted. White is
very high; dark is very low. So this tug of war on your body
creates stress that must be released by spring's light, fresh
green through the release of toxins built up in the tissues due to
pollution, home heating units, poor food supply. Enjoy your
North land! There are tools at every corner to help you thrive in
these climates. The world was designed so!*

*Now to the matter of earth, that is "dirt". It is full of microbes
that work endlessly to digest harmful bacteria. You must honour
this "dirt" as you call it, as it is the sustainer of your physical
being. Honour sand! Honour humus! Honour clay! All have their
precious microbes that lend their part in keeping this earth
space clear of invasion by parasites, fungi and harmful bacteria
and microbes. These would take hold and be rampant on your
earth-more so than now- but for the earth!*

*Open your eyes to the beauty of "earth". It teems with life if no
pesticides are dumped on it. You kill this teeming life with your
pesticides and herbicides, your residues, your toxic wastes!
Open up to the beauty of the earth. It is there for a reason. The
reason is your very sustenance. You are killing the very microbes
that that can eliminate the viruses, the flu bugs, the pandemics
you so fear. Open your eyes to what beauty lies in "dirt".
Rename it to a name that elevates its' status in your eyes to
that which shall be honoured and revered. For in doing that,
then you will resolve your fears of devastation, of pandemics.*

Indeed such a future awaits if you do not cease with the destruction of these precious microbes by your "chemical" saviors - so-called.

Now to the matter of mowing lawns. Yes, you may wish to cut the grass so it looks less runaway or wild. However, as you do this you are also releasing spores from the earth every time you run over the organisms that produce these spores. So mow your lawns at the dewy time to keep the transmission of these spores of fungus to a minimum. Do not chose a dry time as this causes further distribution to your neighbours' lot. I know this is a fun pastime for you - this mowing of lawns -with all your ride-ons, etc. But mow less frequently to promote more energy around your houses and to minimize the transmission of these spores in the air.

I cannot stress enough that as the body attempts to move upward in frequency it will need all the help it can get by way of cutting down its detractors, that is excess fungal spores, and by increasing its helpers, more high frequency producing plants and foods.

YOUR SELF-CLEANING SYSTEM

I turn your attention to a specifically important function in the human body. I will address its' wellness through the use of specific foods. This is the function of lymphatic drainage in the body. To perform this incredible cleansing function in your body it is necessary for the body to have specific tools in place. Just as a carpenter cannot build a dazzling Taj Mahal with only a saw, neither can your body build the magnificence that is the design of the physical body.

Let us begin with an understanding of the lymphatic system. This is your "central vac" system. Its' job is to clean every nook and cranny of your body millions of times. As workmen must constantly sweep and polish the main thoroughfares of your cities and towns so too must the lymphatic system sweep, brush, mop, shovel sometimes, the debris, the gunk, the sticky residues that collect in your body daily.

This is no easy chore due to the poor food supply, your air quality, your noise pollution, your Extremely Low Frequencies, your rush and hurry lives, your sleepless nights! These all contribute to overload, to excess debris, to tired, overworked carpenters, shall I say, manning the brooms, the mops, the scrub brushes. You are all at risk on this one! The lymphatic system is the starting point of our journey with you back to wellness- wellness individually and wellness collectively. For as you raise your states of bring, you raise the very state, of the planet!

The lymphatic system's task is much facilitated by the selection of foods which by their nature have a cleansing and sweeping action. The family of foods that are of that particular nature are the citrus fruits - lemons, limes, oranges, grapefruits, and kiwi. Though not citrus, I also mention pineapple and cantaloupe in this family of cleaning helpers that sweep debris from the body.

The preparation of these fruits before their ingestion is very important. They are by nature highly acidic - thereby pungent and biting to the taste buds. To soften their effect, sprinkle iodized sea salt over them before consuming.

I recommend the ingestion of three helpings of these fruits every day for at least four weeks. During this time you may see marked changes in your bodily routine. That is your urination and bowel movements will increase remarkably. This is the body cleaning itself out, shoveling the debris to the exits shall I say!

You must remember the balanced ion state of your water is of the utmost importance in this process. Now to the use of these fruits in your menus. These may be introduced into salads, supper dishes, cakes, even cookies.

What follows are four special recipes to stimulate your creative uses of these products. You will see how easy it will be to incorporate these prepared fruits into your bodies to do the work they were designed to do.

FRUIT SALAD #1

1 cup shredded red cabbage
1 cup cantaloupe, diced
1 cup pineapple, diced
1 cup carrots

Dressing:
1 t. nutmeg
1 T. yogurt
1 T. honey
1 t. paprika

Pour dressing over fruit and vegetables. Then add:
1 cup crushed walnuts
1 T. coconut

FRUIT SALAD #2:

1 cup oranges
1 cup grapefruit
1 cup unsweetened coconut
1 T. walnuts crushed

<u>*Dressing:*</u>
1 t. iodized sea salt
¼ t. almond extract
1 cup yogurt

Toss together and serve.

FRUIT SALAD #3:

1 avocado peeled and diced
1 pear processed diced
1 cup oranges, diced
1 cup pineapple, diced
1 granny smith apple - grated, skin on

<u>*Dressing:*</u>
1 T. sunflower oil
1 T. olive oil
1 T. walnut oil
1 t. cinnamon
1 t. nutmeg
1 egg beaten
1 T. umeboshi vinegar
1 t. iodized sea salt.

Pour dressing over, sprinkle with 1 T. sunflower seeds.

COOKIES:

1 cup coconut
1 cup cocoa
1 T. honey
1 T. dates chopped
1 T. raw sugar cane
1 cup oranges, pureed
1 T. hazelnut oil or olive oil
1 cup spelt
1 t. baking soda
1 t. baking powder
1 T. sunflower oil
1 T. olive oil
1 T. butter
1 t. peppermint extract
1 cup yogurt

Combine spelt, coconut, cocoa, dates, baking soda and baking powder
Combine remaining ingredients. Then incorporate the dry ingredients into the wet ingredients. Place bowl on the North side of a magnet for 10 min. Drop by spoonful on a prepared baking sheet. Bake at 350 degrees, 15-20 minutes.

FAST FOOD FACTS

SPELT FLOUR- This flour is used because its' balanced, high ion content, means it takes much less spelt in cookies, cakes to create a flavourful, easily digested product.

FLAX SEED- It imparts more value to the body, nutrient wise, when crushed and added to baked goods than when sprouted and used in salads.

SWEETENERS- Raw Sugar cane is balanced in negative and positive ions. When harvested by hand even more negative ions are retained.

HONEY- is the best choice as it is 100% in balance with respect to the negative and positive ions. Raw sugar cane is 90% in balance and molasses is 50%. I would also mention that maple syrup is 80 % in balance. However when you cook with honey you lose 50% of the negative ions so use honey raw or add at the end of the cooking time where possible. Both molasses and sugar cane remain stable in cooking.

RICE- Grown in water fields. Basmati rice, harvested by hand retains 80% of its negative ions. When you cook it with 1 t. of turmeric per ½ cup of precooked rice plus 1 t. of sunflower oil and ½ t. iodized salt, you increase the negative ions to 100%. Combining cooked basmati rice with diced pickled peppers enhances the release of nutrients from both items. Adding cooked basmati rice to potatoes in their skins, cubed, along with ½ cup parsley, and ½ t. of lemon juice releases more nutrients from the potato and makes the starches of both the rice and the potato more digestible.

NOTE! Combining rice with milk negates the nutrients of each other. Wrong combination!!

MILK PRODUCTS- Plain, cultured yogurt and fresh fruit: Dice up 3 kinds of fruit (leave skins on nectarines, plums, peaches) add to 8 oz. yogurt and 1 T. of non pasteurized honey. Let stand for

10 min. This slight fermentation causes the release of otherwise unavailable nutrients from the fruit.

CHEESE - Raw cheese has more enzymes. Enzymes attract negative ions. This is also why it is important to eat cheese with fruit and wine. Brie, havarti, parmesan, old white cheddar (from raw milk) and Gouda are good choices. Heating milk diminishes the negative ions,

YOGOURT: Do add fresh fruit as noted previously. However do not add the alcohol-fermented fruit as the absorption of the iron in the fruit is inhibited by the fat.

MEATS- Processed meats are low in negative ions. Properly prepared raw meats are the best source. There are ways to cook meats that keep the negative ion count higher. They are:
- In water plus iodized sea salt.
- Use rice cooked in turmeric, iodized sea salt and sunflower oil as the stuffing.
- Braise quickly on high heat then cover and simmer in 1 T. water per 2 oz. of meat.
- Barbeque-fast cooking at a high heat, but marinade before hand at least 10 minute and only add sauces at the last minute.

Suggested marinades:
- Beef per pound-1 T. vinegar (red wine or umboshi), 1 T. olive oil, seasonings.
- Chicken per pound - 1 T. lemon juice, 1 T. sunflower oil, seasonings.
- Pork per pound- 1 T. vinegar (red wine or umboshi), 1 T. canola oil, seasonings.
- Seafood, fish – 1 T. lemon juice, 1 T. sunflower oil, seasonings.

Seasonings that are high in negative ions:
- For Beef- curry, turmeric, garlic, onion.
- For Chicken- curry, honey, mustard, cloves, ginger, cinnamon, miso, dill, tarragon, rosemary, chives, garlic, tomato paste, anchovy sauce, oyster sauce.

- *For Pork: Tamarind sauce, ginger, cinnamon, salt/pepper, garlic, mint, cloves, garlic, parsley, onion, black pepper.*
- *For Seafood-lemon, chives, dill, tarragon, parsley, cilantro, rose petals, mint, basil, thyme, oregano.*

BEANS-
> *Kidney beans - for riboflavin*
> *Navy beans – calcium*
> *Pinto beans - magnesium*
> *Black beans - selenium*
> *Lima beans - cobalt*

Special considerations:
Kidney beans should be cooked with tomatoes - canned or fresh.
Navy beans- for 1 cup of beans add 1 T. balsamic vinegar and 1 T. olive oil.
Pinto beans-When serving add 1 T. sunflower oil per cup of cooked beans.

BUTTER- Unsalted butter is not a good choice in the diet as you require the addition of the iodine in salt to transport the fat throughout the digestive system. However, most butters are salted with common table salt. So purchase unsalted if you can not find butter with iodized sea salt. For table use add ½ t. iodized sea salt to 1 cup of softened butter. In a recipe for each ½ cup of butter, add ¼ t. of salt.

Note: if there is no iodized salt added when using butter, coconut oil or sunflower oil, they will not break down to transport nutrients. If this is the case they are then stored as cholesterol in the body.

FERMENTED FOODS- The value of slight fermentation of fruits and vegetables is the release of vitamins and minerals bound up in the fruit, vegetable or grain not otherwise available to the body. It is the chlorophyll that is broken down so the nutrients can be released.

For carrots, ginger, brussel sprouts, squash, radishes, green or yellow beans
(blanche beans in boiling water 5 minutes before processing):

Fill one glass quart jar to the top with the sliced vegetables. Add 1 T. iodized sea salt, and 1 T. plain, cultured yogourt. Fill the jar to the top with your ionized water. Tighten a lid on the jar. Leave the jar sitting on the counter top for 4 days. Use on the fifth day as required. Refrigerate the jar of vegetables after opening.

For fruits such as pineapple, pears, nectarines, plums, peaches, grapes, apples, cantaloupe and melons: clean the fruit that the skins l remain on (i.e. pears, nectarines, apples and grapes, plums) by immersing in water with 1 T. white natural vinegar for 10 minutes. Drain. Peel the pineapple, cantaloupe and melons. Remove seeds and dice. Fill a 1 quart glass jar with the prepared fruit. Fill to the top with a mixture of 1 part vodka to 4 parts ionized water. Tighten lid on jar and place it in a dark cupboard for 3 days. Begin using on the fourth day and refrigerate thereafter.

For berries - strawberries, raspberries, blueberries follow the same procedure but use the following to ferment: 1 part white wine ("0" in sweetness) to 3 parts ionized water.

NUTS and OILS –
Brazil Nuts contain potassium and calcium ash essential to the uptake of zinc. The calcium ash also helps maintain the acid/alkaline balance in the body.
Almonds contain oleic acid. The best way to prepare almonds: grind up ½ cup of skinless almonds. Add 1 T. lemon juice to make a paste. Let sit for 10 minutes. Add 1 T. to breads, muffins, cakes, biscuits before baking. Or spread on a slice of bread as a snack.

***NOTE: It is important to have an enzyme-rich diet when consuming nuts (i.e. add in avocados, raw cheeses, yogourt).

Almond oil can be heated up in cooking the same as olive oil. It is wise to vary your use of these two oils, alternating between the two. Almond extract is high in cobalt. Try to use ¼ t. in all baked goods. Almond extract or peppermint extract plus butter eliminates the caffeine in ground coffee beans when left to soak for 10 minutes.

Walnuts contain linoleic acid. This delicious dressing scores a 10 on the ionized chart due to the combination of crushed walnuts and sunflower oil.

  1 T. sunflower oil
  1 T. olive oil
  1 T. balsamic vinegar
  1 T. crushed walnuts
  1 T. crushed flax seed
  1 T. Italian seasoning or Oregano

Shake together, let sit 10 minutes to combine flavours.

Sunflower Oil contains oleic acid. Sunflower oil combined with olive oil increases the liver's ability to take up nutrients by 100%!!

SUNFLOWER MAYONNAISE

1 T. sunflower oil
1 cup cultured yogourt
1 T. honey
1 T. vinegar
1 t. mustard
1/4 t. iodized sea salt
2 T. grapeseed oil
1 T. crushed walnuts
¼ t. paprika
¼ t. turmeric
1 egg

Mix well together in blender.

Coconut oil contains linoleic acid. When combined with butter, 1 T. butter and 1 T. coconut oil, the synergy creates the best source of Vitamin A and D.

OLIVE OIL - Always use 100% pure virgin olive oil in dark coloured bottles. One T. olive oil plus 1 T. lemon juice will enhance the body's absorption of Vitamin C. One T. olive oil with fresh or frozen corn releases Vitamin D.

CANOLA OIL- Do not use canola oil for frying. When you combine canola oil with olive oil, Vitamins P and K are produced synergistically. Canola oil with nuts such as almond, brazil, walnuts releases calcium.

GINGER - should be grated fresh, then lacto-fermented. This ensures that valuable nutrients are released and available to the body. Ginger is the best source for folic acid in the plant and animal kingdom. This is very valuable-inestimable in fact- in face of the rapid decline of folic acid in the body due to present dietary conditions, and due to the stress the body experiences in these ever increasing frequencies. So eat ginger bread, ginger cookies, drink ginger tea!! Go ahead... over-consume ginger. It is a gift to you!!

KITCHEN STAPLES

sesame seeds
flax seeds
sunflower seeds
walnuts
pecans
almonds
olive oil
sesame seed oil
grapeseed oil
coconut oil
canola oil
raw sugar cane
honey
molasses
corn syrup
iodized sea salt
canned water chestnuts
canned sardines
cornmeal
spelt
arrowroot flour
cinnamon sticks

dried ginger
turmeric
paprika
whole nutmeg
bay leaves
whole black pepper
lemon juice
quinoa
curry powder
raisins
dates
figs
coconut
lard
butter
bean sauce
fish sauce
red lentils
hot chili sauce
tomato sauce
basmati rice
long grain white rice

BREAKFAST RECIPES

PANCAKES

Overnight, soak:
1 cup oatmeal
1 cup water
1 T. lemon juice

In the morning add:
2 cups buttermilk / yogourt
1 T. butter
1 T. sunflower oil / grape seed oil
¼ cup raw sugar cane
2 eggs
1 T. cinnamon
1 T. chopped walnuts
1 T. ground flax seeds
¼ cup spelt
½ t. baking soda
½ t. baking powder
¼ cup corn (frozen or fresh)
¼ cup parmesan cheese
¼ cup raisins
¼ cup chopped dates
1 banana, mashed

*Sift dry ingredients. Incorporate into the wet ingredients.
Heat a cast iron skillet until water droplets dance on the
surface, then heat 1 t. olive oil. Drop batter by the spoonful on
skillet to cook.*

CREPES

1 egg
1 T. milk
½ cup spelt
1 T. crushed walnuts
1 T. ground flax seeds
1 T. butter

Cook in a preheated cast iron skillet in 1 T. olive oil.
Stuff with shrimp, tomato, diced dill pickle, 1 T. yogourt, salt &
pepper. Drizzle with sunflower oil.

GRANOLA

Prepare "CORNMEAL BISCUIT" recipe. Roll to ½" thick and bake
according to directions. Crumble when cool. Add:
1 cup chopped walnuts
1 cup chopped almonds
1 cup sesame seeds
1 cup ground flax seeds

Toss together and toast in oven for 1 hour at 325, watch closely
and turn half way through. When cooled, add:
1 cup raisins
1 cup chopped dates
 1 T. cinnamon
1 t. nutmeg
1 T. sunflower oil

Store in an airtight container.

COCONUT CEREAL

1 cup unsweetened coconut
1 cup milk / whey
1 T. walnuts
1 T. arrowroot flour
1 t. cinnamon
1 T. honey / raw sugar cane
1 T. dates
1 T. raisins
1 T. butter

Heat for 5 minutes, but do not allow mixture to boil. Serve as a breakfast cereal.

BREAKFAST CEREAL

1 cup cornmeal
2 cups hot water
Salt to taste
1 t. cinnamon
1 T. ground flaxseed
1 T. crushed walnuts
2 T. raisins
2 T. chopped dates
1 t. sunflower oil

Combine ingredients and bring to a boil. Reduce heat and stir for 5 minutes.
Serve with yogurt and honey, or use in pancake recipe that follows.

CEREAL PANCAKES

1 cup cooked cereal (see previous recipe)
1 egg
½ t. baking soda
½ t. baking powder
2 T. raw sugar cane
1 T. raisins
½ cup spelt
2 T. olive oil
1 T. butter

Soak the following ingredients for 10 minutes:
½ cup buttermilk
½ cup crushed fresh pineapple
½ t. red wine vinegar

Add to cereal mixture and cook in a preheated cast iron skillet lightly coated with olive oil.

PORRIDGE

½ cup oatmeal
2 cups water
1 t. lemon juice
Combine above ingredients and place on the north side of a magnet for 10 minutes.

Add:
1 T. ground flax seed
1 T. crushed sunflower seeds
1 T. cinnamon
1 t. salt
1 T. sunflower oil

Add fruit of choice: Raisins, apple, figs, dates. Cook for 10 minutes over medium heat.

LEFTOVER PORRIDGE PANCAKES

2 cups cooked porridge (see previous recipe)

<u>Add</u>:
1 egg
½ cup spelt
1 t. baking soda
1 t. baking powder
1 T. raw sugar cane T. raisins
2 T. olive oil
1 T. butter
½ cup buttermilk/yogourt

Drop by spoonful on a preheated cast iron skillet lightly oiled with olive oil.

LUNCH / DINNER RECIPES

BBQ'D HAMBURGERS

2 lbs. ground beef
1 T. hot chilies, chopped
1 T. chopped parsley
1 T. molasses
1 T. Italian seasoning
1 T. butter
1 T. beer
2 T. bread crumbs

Assemble ingredient and let sit for 10 minutes o the north side
of a magnet.
Form into patties, and grill or broil.

HAMBURGER BUNS

2 cups spelt
1 T. yeast
1 T. whey or yogourt
1 t. salt
1 t. vinegar
½ cup sourdough starter or yogourt
1 t. baking soda
2 cups beer

Add yeast to whey and sourdough starter plus vinegar for 10
minutes on north side of a magnet.

Add baking soda to spelt, then add spelt to yeast mixture. Add beer. Knead and let rise for 20 minutes. Form into buns. Let rise for another 20 minutes.
Bake at 400 for 10-15 minutes.

TACOS AND BEANS

<u>Mash together</u>:
2 cups cooked navy beans
2 cups cooked (in skins) cubed potatoes

<u>Add</u>:
2 T. sunflower oil
2 T. olive oil
1 T. balsamic vinegar
1 T. Italian seasoning
2 T. tomato sauce
1 ½ t. salt

Heat 6 corn tortilla shells and fill with:
Bean mixture
1 cup yogourt
1 cup diced tomatoes
1 cup diced cucumber
Hot pickled peppers, chopped
1 cup fermented carrots

Top with shredded cheese and parsley. Place upright in a cast iron skillet in a 350 degree oven for 10-15 minutes. Sprinkle with crushed walnuts before serving.

PORK AND NOODLES

1 lb. pork filet, sliced diagonally
<u>Marinate in:</u>
½ cup olive oil
1 T. tandoori powder or paste

<u>Chop:</u>
1 cup bok choy
1 cup green onion
1 cup tomato
1 cup green beans

Sauté meat. Remove from heat then sauté vegetables. Soften 2 cups egg noodles in hot water, then drain.
Combine meat, vegetables and noodles. Add 2 T. bean sauce and serve.

RED LENTILS

1 green onion, chopped
1 cup red lentils
2 cups water

Soak above ingredients for 10 minutes on the north side of a magnet. Then add:
1 small zucchini, chopped
1 carrot chopped
½ t. salt

Cook for 20 minutes, then add:
1 cup cooked rice
1 cup cooked potato (in skins) cubed
1 cup tomato sauce
1 T. grated ginger, or 1 t. powdered ginger
1 T. cinnamon
1 T. sunflower oil

WHITE BEANS (NAVY BEANS)

2 cups cooked beans
½ cucumber, diced
2 T. tomato sauce
½ T. lemon juice
1 cup cooked ham, cubed
1 cup cooked basmati rice
1 T. sunflower oil
Salt / pepper / cayenne

WHITE BEANS (2)

2 cups cooked white beans
1 cup lacto fermented carrots
1 cup lacto fermented cucumbers
1 tomato, diced

Sauce:
1 cup yogourt
1 t. nutmeg
1 t. cinnamon
1 T. olive oil
1 T. sunflower oil
salt

Fill a taco shell with bean mixture. Top with sauce and grated cheese.

BLACK BEANS

2 cups cooked back beans
1 T. sunflower oil
2 T. tomato sauce
1 cup diced water chestnuts
1 t. cumin

1 T. walnuts, crushed
Cook above ingredients.

Serve with basmati rice cooked with:
1 t. turmeric, 1/2 t. iodized sea salt, 1 t. sunflower oil
½ onion, diced.Before serving, add ½ cup chopped parsley.

KIDNEY BEANS

2 cups cooked kidney beans
1 T. olive oil
1 T. hot peppers, chopped
½ cup finely chopped kale
1 t. lemon juice

Mix together and serve.

THAI CHICKEN

1 cup water chestnuts
1 cup parsley
1 green onion, diced
1 T. sunflower oil
1 T. olive oil
¼ t. cayenne pepper
1 green pepper, diced
1 raw potato, grated, with skin on
1 boneless, skinless chicken breast
1 T. sesame seeds
1 t. sesame oil
1 cup asparagus

Cook chicken breast in 2 cups water and a dash of salt. Dice.
In a cast iron pan, sauté onion in olive oil. Add green pepper,
potato, asparagus. Steam for 5 minutes. Add chicken plus broth
and remaining ingredients.

Serve over noodles cooked in water with 1 T. fish sauce.
Serve with orange salad.

GUMBO

2 cups beef stock
1 cup lacto-fermented carrots
1 cup cooked potatoes, cubed (skin on)
2 slices cooked ham, sliced into this strips
1 cup cooked basmati rice
1 T. sunflower oil
1 cup uncooked macaroni
1 T. butter
1 T. Italian seasoning
2 T. grated zucchini
1 t. nutmeg
1 t. cinnamon

Cook macaroni in beef stock with butter and sunflower oil.
Do not drain.
Add carrots, potato, rice, ham, zucchini. Heat for 5 minutes.
Add seasonings and serve.

STUFFED TOMATO SUPPER DISH

6 tomatoes, slice off tops, scoop out seeds and pulp, reserve
Mix pulp and seeds with:
1 cup cornmeal or breadcrumbs
1 cup liverwurst sausage, cooked
1 T. Italian seasoning
1 T. butter
1 T. olive oil
Salt / pepper to taste

Stuff tomato with cornmeal mixture. Sprinkle with Gouda
cheese. Bake at 350 for 30 minutes.

SESAME CHICKEN STIR FRY
2 cups boneless chicken, cut in strips
1 T. sesame oil
1 T. olive oil
Marinate above ingredients in a bowl and set on the North side
of a magnet for 10 min.

Combine:
2 zucchini, peeled and sliced diagonally
1 green pepper, diced
1 onion, sliced
1 T. hot chilies, diced

Sauce:
1 T. sesame seeds
1 T. macadamia butter
1 T. soya sauce
1 T. olive oil
1 T. balsamic vinegar

In a cast iron skillet, sauté chicken in oils. Remove from pan and sauté vegetables. Add cooked chicken. Drizzle sauce over and heat through.

HAWAIIAN PASTA

2 pints Hawaiian chutney
1 cup olives
1 cup fresh tomatoes, diced
1 cup green peppers, diced
1 T. miso paste
1 T. olive oil
1 T. sunflower oil
1 T. coconut oil
1 T. coconut
1 T. crushed walnuts
1 T. pine nuts

Mix together. Cook 2 cups pasta in 4 cups water, 1 cup parsley and 1 t. salt.
Drain, and toss with chutney mixture.

TOMATO LUNCHEON PASTA

5 large tomatoes, skins removed, diced
1 large green pepper, seeded and chopped
2 large onions, chopped
1 T. vinegar
1 T. sunflower oil
1 T. crushed cinnamon stick
Salt / pepper to taste.

Simmer above ingredients for 1 hour.

Cook 2 cups penne pasta in 4 cups water, 1 t. lemon juice and 1 cup parsley.
Cook for 10 minutes. Drain.
Add tomato sauce. Sprinkle with feta cheese and 1 T. sunflower oil.

SHRIMP AND SWEET POTATOES

1 T. olive oil
2 cups peeled, cubed sweet potato
1 cup sliced green pepper
½ cup sliced onion
½ cup diced pickled hot chili peppers
1" cube of fresh gingerroot
1 cup green beans
1 orange, peeled and cubed
1 cup bok choy (nappa) sliced diagonally

Heat olive oil, ad all ingredient and stir fry. Add 1 T. fish sauce.

Marinate for 10 min. sitting on North side of a magnet:
¼ cup olive oil
1 T. tandoori powder or paste
25-30 peeled shrimp
 Then cook gently for 5 minutes.
Combine vegetables and shrimp.
Serve over basmati rice mixed with 1 t. turmeric.

SOUFFLE

2 cups sour milk
4 eggs, beaten
1 T. butter
1 T. flour
1 cup grated cheese (gouda or brie)
1 T. olive oil
4 slices stale bread, made into crumbs
1 T. sunflower oil
2 cups fresh spinach
1 T. hot chili peppers (pickled)
1 T. olives, chopped
1 cup lacto fermented carrots
Salt / nutmeg
3 cups chicken stock

Soak breadcrumbs in oils and sour milk for 10 minutes.
Let sit on the north side of a magnet for 10 minutes.
Add eggs, cheese, butter, flour, and pour into a buttered glass baking dish (soufflé dish).
Place in oven along with a container of hot water. Bake at 375 for 30 minutes. Use buttered brown paper to extend height of soufflé dish if necessary. Serve with fresh spinach, chilies, olives, nutmeg, and a drizzle of sunflower oil.

SOUP COMBINATIONS

CARROTS AND POTATO
2 carrots, chopped fine
2 potatoes, chopped fine

Heat to sweat vegetables in 1 T. olive oil and 1 T. butter and 2 T. water for 10 minutes in a covered stainless steel pot.
Add: 4 oz. whey (milk / buttermilk / yogourt) and 12 oz. water.
Cook 10 minutes longer. Puree with hand beater.

Add:
1 T. sunflower oil
1 T. dried basil, or 2 T. fresh basil
Salt & pepper to taste

Heat through and serve.

ONION AND PARSNIP SOUP

Prepare as above, using onions and parsnip in place of carrot and potato.
At the end, use Italian seasoning in place of basil.

KALE SOUP

Prepare as above, using 2 cups shredded kale in place of carrots and potatoes.
Add juice of ½ lemon before serving.

GREEN PEPPER AND SQUASH SOUP

1 green pepper, chopped fine
Heat and sweat in 2 T. olive oil. Add whey and water (as above).

Add 1 cup cooked squash
1 T. Italian seasoning
1 T. cinnamon

BEAN SOUP

½ cup diced green pepper
½ cup onion, chopped

Heat and sweat in 1 T. olive oil and 1 T. butter.

Add:
2 cups cooked white beans
1 T. miso paste
1 cup whey (yogourt) plus 3 cups water
1 T. Italian seasoning

Heat through and serve.

SHRIMP FROM ANOTHER DIMENSION

24-30 raw shrimp, shelled, marinated for 10 mins. in:
- 1 t. tandoori powder or paste
- ¼ cold pressed, extra virgin olive oil

Then sauté shrimp with:
- 1 T. green onion, grated
- 1 T. green pepper, chopped
- 1 T. carrot, grated
- 1 T. hot chilies, chopped
- 1 T. walnuts, chopped

Meanwhile, prepare basmati rice: two cups hot water, 1 cup of basmati rice with 1 T. turmeric and 1 T. sunflower oil and 1 t. iodized sea salt. Combine the shrimp mixture with the rice, and add juice of 1 lime, 1 T sunflower oil or grapeseed oil.

CHICKEN SOUP (REALLY FOR THE SOUL)

Sweat in olive oil in large covered, stainless steel pot:
1 kolrabi
1 potato-unpeeled
1 large carrot
1 green onion
2 cloves garlic
1 cup frozen green beans

Fill to ½ full with water. Add chicken carcass, salt, dash of vinegar. Simmer 2 hours. Just before serving, add parsley, 1 T. butter, 1 T. Italian seasoning.

ROAST CHICKEN

Stuff chicken with mixture of:
2 cups basmati rice, cooked with 1 T. turmeric and 1 T.
sunflower oil, salt to taste
1 T. Italian seasoning
1 chopped onion

Roast at 350 F for two hours, in an open pan.

BEVERAGE RECIPES

COFFEE FOR TWO *(sans caffeine!)*

1 T. ground chicory coffee beans or beans of choice
1 t. hazelnut oil
1 t. peppermint oil
1 t. butter

Let sit for 10 minutes on the north side of a magnet.
Add 16 oz. boiling water and serve.

DECAFFINATED COFFEE

¼ t. almond extract
1 t. hazelnut oil
1 t. ground coffee beans
¼ t. butter

Let sit for 10 minutes on the north side of a magnet.
Add 8 oz. hot water and 1 T. whipping cream.

MINERAL DRINK *(for sleep)*

1 cup whey
1 t. cinnamon
1 t. lemon juice

COFFEE ALMOND LATTE

1 t. finely ground coffee
¼ t. almond extract (organic)
1 oz. hot water
4 oz. hot milk
1 t. butter
Set on the north side of the magnet for 10 min.
Serve with a dollop of whipped cream.

IONIZED MINERAL DRINK
(To restore the body's mineral stores, drink 1 serving per day)

2 oz. whey
4 oz. water
1 ½ t. honey
½ t. salt

ION and ENZYME DRINK

1 T. fish sauce,
8 oz water
Enjoy 1 drink per day to restore ion and enzyme levels in the body.

MORNING WAKE-UP DRINK

1 t. sesame seed oil
1 T. raw sugar cane
1 t. instant coffee
2 oz. boiling water
Mix together and add 6 oz. yogourt.

MORNING WAKE-UP DRINK #2

1 cup thawed berries (strawberries, raspberries, ore blueberries) mashed
1 T. sunflower oil
1 T. honey / raw sugar cane
6 oz. yogourt

CINNAMON TEA

2 sticks of cinnamon
1 whole clove
¼ t. honey
¼ t. butter
1/8 t. iodized sea salt
8 oz water Simmer 10 min
High in selenium, vanadium, chromium, cobalt and copper. You can drink it 3 times a day!

KIWI TEA

1 peeled kiwi mashed
¼ t. honey
¼ t. butter
1/8 t. iodized sea salt
8 oz. boiling water
Simmer 10 mins.
High in chromium, selenium, germanium and choline.

STRAWBERRY TEA

4 crushed field strawberries
¼ t. honey
1 t. cinnamon
Dash nutmeg
8 oz. water
Simmer 10 min.
Contains vitamins C, D, P, K, and iron.

CITRUS TEA

1 cup peeled oranges/ grapefruit/lemon/ or pineapple
¼ t. honey
¼ t. butter
1 t. cinnamon, dash nutmeg
Simmer 10 min.
Sieve and serve.
Contains Vitamins P, K, and riboflavin

NUTMEG TEA

1 nutmeg grated
¼ t. honey
¼ t. butter
1 t. vanilla
8 oz water
Simmer 10 mins.
Contains chromium, cobalt, silicon, and germanium.

GREEN TEA ENHANCEMENT

1 green tea bag
Juice of 1 lime
1 t. honey
The addition of the lime is for Vitamin C, but the combination creates the frequency of Vitamin D. Honey added provides the enzymes to bind with the minerals. Green tea contains zinc, chromium, vanadium, selenium and cobalt

DESSERT RECIPES

PARFAIT

2 cups whipped cream
Add:
½ cup crushed walnuts
1 T. cocoa
1 t. finely ground coffee, pre-soaked in 1 t. almond oil and 1 t. butter for 10 min.
1 egg, slightly beaten

Add 1 cup ricotta cheese
*Brandied fruit of choice-see directions

Layer ricotta mixture, then brandied fruit in a parfait glass. Repeat layers. Garnish with chocolate shavings, cocoa, or brandied fruit.

FRUIT DESSERT

Slice 2 bananas or oranges

Sprinkle with:
1 T. honey
1 T. raw sugar cane
1 T. crushed walnuts or pecans or coconut (or all three)
1 t .cinnamon

Drizzle with sunflower oil and grated nutmeg.
Place under broiler for 2 minutes.

"GO" BAR

1 T. honey
1 T. sesame seeds
1 T. whipping cream
1 T. butter
1 T. sunflower oil
1 T. chopped dates
1 T. chopped raisins
2 oz. unsweetened chocolate
½ t. almond extract
1 T. molasses
1 T. coconut oil
2 T. cocoa
2 T. unsweetened coconut
3 T. each: crushed flax seeds, sunflower seeds, walnuts
1/2 cup arrowroot flour
1 T. hazelnut oil

Combine and press into pan. Bake at 325 for 25 minutes.
Consume 3-1" bars a day for "Go" power!!

PEANUT BUTTER COOKIES   (or ALMOND or MACADAMIA)

1 cup nut butter
½ cup raw sugar cane
½ cup butter
1 t. lemon juice
½ t. salt
¼ cup spelt
1 egg
1 t. baking soda
1 cup raisins (or dates, or figs, or unsweetened coconut, or chocolate chips)

Drop by the teaspoonful onto baking sheet. Bake at 350 for 12 minutes.

MAPLE SYRUP DELIGHT

5 eggs, separated:
Whip egg whites until stiff
Cream yolks with ½ t. lemon juice plus 1 T. raw sugar cane

Mix: ½ cup spelt
1 cup cocoa
1 t. baking soda

Combine: 1 T. sunflower oil with 1 T. butter, 1/2 cup maple syrup and add to the spelt/chocolate mixture

In small amounts, combine egg yolk mixture and spelt / butter mixture. Fold in the beaten egg whites.

Crush 5 chocolate wafer biscuits in the bottom of a springform pan, cover with half of cake mixture. Crush 5 more biscuits on top, then remaining cake mixture. On top drizzle a combination of 1 T. hazelnut oil and ½ cup crushed walnuts. Bake at 350 for 30 minutes.

CHOCOLATE CHIPS

½ cup cocoa
1 oz unsweetened chocolate
1 T. butter
1 T. raw sugar cane
1 T. coconut oil
1 T. corn syrup
1 T. water
1 T. whipping cream
1 t. vanilla

Combine in the top of a double boiler, cook for 10 min. Pour onto a buttered piece of wax paper. Place in refrigerator. When hard break into small pieces.

WORLD'S BEST CHOCOLATE CHIP COOKIES!!

<u>Cream together</u>:
½ cup butter
½ cup coconut oil
½ cup raw sugar cane

Add 2 eggs.

<u>Sift together</u>:
1 cup oatmeal
1 cup unsweetened coconut
11/4 cup spelt flour
1 t. baking soda
1 t. baking powder
1 T. cocoa
1 t. nutmeg
1 t. cinnamon
Chocolate chips (see recipe above)

Add dry ingredients to wet ingredients. Bake at 350 for 12-15 minutes.

PMS COOKIES

¼ cup cream
1 cup cocoa
2 T. corn syrup
2 T. butter
1 cup unsweetened coconut

½ cup chopped pecans
1 T. sunflower oil
1/4 cup spelt
1 t. baking soda
1 egg
1 t. vanilla

Drop by the spoonful onto baking sheet. Bake at 350 for 12 minutes.

BROWNIES

Melt together:
2 squares unsweetened chocolate
½ cup butter
½ cup cream

Mix together:
2 eggs
 1 ½ t. baking soda
½ cup raw sugar cane
½ cup cocoa
½ cup chopped walnuts
1 T. sunflower seeds
1 T. ground flax seeds
1 T. sunflower oil
1 peeled avocado mashed

Add mixture to melted chocolate mixture. Pour into a prepared cake pan.
Bake at 350 for 30 mins.

ICE CREAM

2 cups whipping cream (not whipped)
½ cup raw sugar cane or honey
2 eggs
1 kiwi or other fruit, chopped
1 T. lime juice
Use ice cream maker, or freeze in a shallow dish

BRANDIED FRUIT

1 part brandy, 4 parts water
Leave peel on fruit. Dice your choice of pear, plum, nectarine, cherries, peaches.
If using peaches, peel them. Pack fruit into glass jar, cover with brandy mixture. Store in a dark place for 4 days. Refrigerate after opening.

FERMENTED CITRUS FRUIT

Slice and dice 2 oranges plus 1 grapefruit
Place together in a quart jar.
Add 1 part vodka to 4 parts ionized water to fill jar to top-fruit covered.
Store in a cool dark place for 4 days. Use 1 T. fruit in yogurt or over ice cream. Refrigerate after opening.

DEVINE CHOCOLATE CAKE with CHOCOLATE SAUCE

Melt:
2 squares unsweetened chocolate
1 T. butter
Add: 1 cup buttermilk (or yogourt)

Sift:
1 ½ cups spelt flour
1 t. baking powder
1 t. baking soda
1 T. cocoa
1 t. cinnamon
1 cup unsweetened coconut

Cream:
½ cup butter with ½ cup coconut oil and ½ cup raw sugar cane
Add 2 eggs.

Alternately in small amounts, add chocolate mixture and dry
ingredients to butter mixture, stirring to blend. Bake at 350 F,
for 45 minutes.

CHOCOLATE SAUCE

Melt 2 squares unsweetened chocolate in a double boiler. Add 1
can evaporated milk.

Whip until a pudding-like texture. Pour over cake. Sprinkle with
pecans, walnuts or coconut.

COCONUT CAKE

<u>Mix:</u>
1 t. lemon juice
1 cup unbleached flour
1 cup buttermilk, or sour milk
½ cup sourdough, if available

<u>Sift:</u>
½ cup spelt
1 T. ground flax seed
1 T. ground sunflower seeds
1 t. baking powder
1 t. baking soda

<u>Cream:</u>
1 cup butter, or 1 cup coconut oil plus 1 T. sunflower oil
½ cup raw sugar cane or honey

Broil 1 cup unsweetened coconut until golden. Watch carefully! Add coconut to sifted ingredients, then alternately and in small amounts, add coconut mixture and buttermilk mixture to the creamed mixture.

Stir in ½ cup chopped dates.
Bake at 350 F, for 45-60 minutes.

EASY ICING

2 T. ground flax seed cooked in ½ cup water until gelatin forms. Cool completely.

Add ½ t. lemon juice, sprinkle of salt
Beat until stiff peaks form.
Add 2 T. raw sugar cane
1 t. vanilla extract

CHOCOLATE BARK

In a double boiler, cook until heated through:
3 T. coconut oil
1 T. butter
1 ½ to 3 T. cocoa (to taste)
¼ cup raw sugar cane+ 1 T. honey
1 T. cream
½ cup almonds, or walnuts or coconut
½ t. vanilla
Dash of cinnamon

Spread thinly on buttered waxed paper. Place in freezer until solid enough to break into pieces. Enjoy!

BREADS/ MUFFINS/ BISCUIT RECIPES

BREAD

Combine and place over the north side of a magnet for 10 min.:
2 cup spelt plus 1 t. baking soda
½ cup sourdough starter
¼ cup cornmeal
2 T. olive oil
2 T. sunflower oil
1 T. butter
1 ¼ cup whey / milk / yogourt
1 T. honey
1 T. iodized sea salt

Combine and place over the North side of a magnet for 10 min.:
2 cups unbleached white flour
2 cup warm water
1 T. lemon juice
1 T. yeast
1 t. honey

<u>Combine:</u>
5 cups spelt
½ cup raisins / dates
1 egg
½ cup crushed walnuts
½ cup ground flax seed
½ cup sunflower seeds

Add sourdough mixture to yeast mixture. Let rise 30 minutes. Place on the North side of a magnet. Add remaining spelt and ingredients. Shape into three round loaves, rub tops with olive oil. Let rise for another 30 minutes. Bake at 375 for 45-55 minutes.

BAKING SODA BISCUITS

Combine:
½ cup unbleached white flour
1 ¼ cup buttermilk / milk / whey
1 T. lemon juice
Let mixture sit for 10 minutes on the north side of a magnet.

Sift together:
1½ cups spelt flour
½ cup arrowroot flour
2 t. baking powder
1 t. baking soda
¼ cup butter
¼ cup sunflower oil

Cut in butter and oil.
Add wet ingredients to dry ingredients.
Optional: Add ¼ cup grated cheese.

Bake at 400 for 15-20 minutes.

CORNMEAL BISCUITS

1 ¼ cup cornmeal
¾ cup spelt flour
1 t. baking soda
1 cup buttermilk
1 T. butter
1 T. sunflower oil
1 T. parmesan cheese
1 T. crushed walnuts

Mix ingredients together. Place on the north side of a magnet for 10 minutes.

Roll out to a 1" thickness. Bake in one piece on a baking sheet, 400 for 15 minutes.
Cut into fingers sized strips for serving.
MAPLE BANANA MUFFINS

Combine:
2 eggs
½ cup butter or coconut oil (or a blend)
1/4 cup raw sugar cane
2 bananas, mashed
½ t. lemon juice
½ cup sourdough starter
!/2 cup pure maple syrup

Combine:
½ cup spelt
½ cup arrowroot
1 t. baking soda
½ t. cinnamon
½ cup crushed pecans
1 T. ground flax seed
1 T. crushed sunflower seeds
Mix wet ingredients with dry ingredients. Drop into prepared muffin tin.

Bake at 350 for 25 minutes.

SOURDOUGH STARTER

2 cups rye flour
2 cups ionized water
½ t. lemon juice
1 t. salt

Leave in a warm place covered with cheesecloth for 3 days.
Start using.

Daily add: ½ cup rye flour plus ½ cup water.
Can store in refrigerator. Bring to room temperature prior to using in recipes.

ORANGE NUT MUFFINS

<u>Combine:</u>
1 ¼ cup spelt
1/2 cup crushed walnuts or pecans
1 T. ground flax seed
1 T. ground sunflower seeds
1 T. cocoa

Combine and place on North side of magnet for 10 min.:
½ cup unbleached white flour
1 T. lemon juice
¾ cup sourdough starter
1 t. baking powder
1 t. baking soda

<u>Cream:</u>
2 eggs
½ cup butter
½ cup raw sugar cane or molasses

<u>Add</u>: 1/2 cup fresh squeezed orange juice
1 T. grated orange rind

Add all the wet ingredients together. Then alternate adding wet to dry ingredients.
Drop mixture by the spoonful into a buttered muffin tin. Bake at 350 degrees for 25 mins.

FLAT BREAD

¼ cup cornmeal
2 cups spelt
1 cup sourdough starter
1 cup whey
1 T. yeast
1 T. honey
1 t. salt
1 T. sunflower oil
1 T. olive oil
1 T. raisins, ground
1 t. cinnamon
¼ t. almond extract

Mix all ingredients together. Then place on North side of magnet for 10 min.
Divide into 10 portions. Roll each out to 1/8" thick, 5" diameter circle. Preheat a heavy cast iron pan at 450 degrees. Place circles of flat bread on hot pan-bake 5 min. per side. These may be stored uncooked in the freezer, between layers of waxed paper, and baked when required.

VEGETABLES/ SALAD RECIPES

OVEN POTATOES

Prepare potatoes by bathing in vinegar bath- leave skins on-
then cut into wedges or cubes
Toss with olive oil
Season with mixture of 1/2 t. cayenne, salt and black pepper.
Bake at 400 F, 25 mins. Turn often.

SEASONED KALE

Pre-soak kale in water with 1 T. vinegar and 1 t. salt
Drain and Pat dry, Then sauté lightly in olive oil for two mins.
Sprinkle with sunflower seeds, and serve

BEETS

2 cups grated raw beets
1 T. lemon juice

Combine and place in a buttered baking dish. Sprinkle with
topping:
1 T. melted butter
1 T. bread crumbs
1 T. crushed walnuts

Bake at 350 for 15-25 minutes until heated through.

EASY DILL PICKLES

Slice cucumbers into long thin slices, leaving seeds in and skins on.
Place in quart jars.

To each jar, add:
- *4 T. whey or 1 T. yogourt*
- *1 T. iodized sea salt*
- *2 sprigs dill*
- *1 clove garlic, crushed (optional)*

Fill to top with water
Seal, leave in cupboard for 4 days, then refrigerate.

Note: Can use whey from yogourt or cottage cheese.

AVOCADO SANDWICH SPREAD

Combine:
1 peeled avocado, mashed
1 t. lemon juice
1 t. balsamic vinegar
1 T. sesame seeds

Puree:
1 nectarine, peeled
1 t. sunflower oil
Combine all the above ingredients. Serve on hardbread, with a piece of endive, lettuce, spinach or radicchio.

ORANGE SALAD

1 orange diced
1 cup fermented carrots
1 T. coconut
1 T. sesame seed oil
1 T. balsamic vinegar
Assemble just before serving

TACO-CADO SALAD

1 avocado, peeled and diced
2 cups endive/spinach
1 apple, diced
1 T. walnuts broken up
1 T. pine nuts
1 T. sesame seeds
1 T sunflower seeds

Dressing:
1 t. sesame seed oil
1 T. sunflower oil
1 T. olive oil
Juice of one orange and one lemon

Toss dressing and salad. Before serving add 1 cup corn tacos broken up.

FAVORITE SALAD

1 avocado peeled and diced
1 orange diced
1 cup raw Kolrabi grated
1 cup strawberries sliced
½ cup parsley

<u>*Dressing:*</u>
1 T olive oil
1 T. honey
1 t. ginger
1 t. yogourt

Toss salad and dressing. Add 1 T. sunflower seeds, 1 T. ground flax seeds, salt and pepper to taste.

ESCAROLE SALAD

1 cup escarole / or raw kale
1 cup lacto fermented carrots
1 T. sunflower oil
1 T. lemon juice
1 T. sesame seeds
1 T. walnuts
1 orange, peeled, sliced and diced

CUCUMBER SALAD

1 cup diced cucumbers
1 cup diced tomatoes
1 T. fish or anchovy sauce
1 T. lemon juice
1 cup parsley chopped
1 T. sesame seeds
1 T. walnuts
1 cup diced cooked chicken

Assemble and toss!

CUCUMBER SALAD #2

1 cucumber peeled and diced
1 T. sunflower oil
1 T. olive oil
1 T. balsamic vinegar
1 T. sunflower seeds
1 T. walnuts

Assemble and toss!

CARROT SALAD

Chop 2 cups lacto fermented carrots
Add:
1 T. sesame seed oil
1 T. sesame seeds
1 T. walnuts
Toss together and serve!

PARSLEY SALAD

1 cup chopped parsley
1 tomato diced
1 green onion diced
1 grapefruit peeled and diced
1 orange peeled and diced
1 T. sunflower seeds
1 t. grape seed oil

Toss and serve!

ENDIVE SALAD

Mix 3 kinds of greens – endive, spinach, radicchio
Add:
1/2 cup water chestnuts, chopped
1 tomato cubed
1 T. walnuts
1 T. ground flax seed
½ cup cubed cheese (Gouda or Brie)

Toss and serve!!

CHEESE AND ASPARAGUS

½ cup parsley
½ avocado peeled and diced
1 cup ricotta cheese
1 pear diced
2 stalks of asparagus, steamed with 1 T. lemon juice for 2 mins.
1 T. flax seed crushed

1 T. sunflower seed oil
½ cup parmesan cheese

Toss and serve!

TOMATO SALSA

Combine in a stainless steel pot and simmer 10 mins:
1 eggplant, peeled and diced.
1 T. iodized sea salt, let soak 10 min. then rinse.
2 lbs. tomatoes - peeled and diced
2 green onions, diced
1 green pepper, diced
1 T. hot peppers
¼ t. cayenne pepper
Pinch of salt
1 banana peeled and mashed
At end of cooking time add:
1 cup lacto fermented carrots
1 T. fresh cilantro
1 cup grated cucumber
1 T. lacto fermented ginger grated
1 clove garlic
1 can sardines chopped up
1 T. olive oil
1 T. sunflower seed oil

SANDWICH SPREAD

1 cup lacto fermented carrots
1 avocado mashed
1 T. sunflower seed oil
1 pear diced
1 T. walnuts crushed
1 T. olive oil

Puree and spread on hard bread.

THE FOURTH DIMENSION

The fourth dimension is a gift to the spirit in human form to know itself in full consciousness as alive in the physical body: to know itself as part of the entire web of creation-no separation, no alienation-only the peace, the joy, the courage to walk into the promised states of love and compassion. This was once known by the spirit in physical, but after the eons, as the frequencies on Mother Earth steadily declined, memory was lost of the wonderment and the childlike, innocent exploration of the physical world- entirely of the soul's own creation. Yes, the collective soul of you all created the original playground, the original human form, the animal forms, even the microbes and the nasty germs!

There was a divine plan at play, and it has now played itself out! It is now the time to return to the memory of why you created this playground and to return to your status, each and every one as creator Gods and Goddesses! As these memories of your great abilities and talents return, you will once again claim the beauty of your journey here. You will begin the re-invention, the re-discovery of the beauty of the plan. Gone will be the anguish, the fears, the lowness of aspiration.

You are capable of solving all that confronts you here on the Earth, for you created this environment in its perfection. You will now find your way back to the wonderment, the awe, the playfulness, the creative expression of your considerable talents! Blessed Be!! You are Gods and Goddesses emerging from your cocoons now in the frequencies of the Fourth Dimension!"

Love,
God, the Creator

BIOGRAPHY

Donna Boynton is a practitioner of Vibrational Medicine as taught by Fabien Mamen, Tama-Do, The Academy of Sound, Colour and Movement. She has studied with Donna Eden, author of 'Energy Medicine'. She resides in New Brunswick, Canada, with her four children. Contact her at:

www.energyflows .com.

Or write to:

Energy Flows
1996 Rothesay Rd.
Rothesay, N.B.
Canada
E2H 2J8